Fighting for King David

Christina Johnson

Copyright © 2018 Christina Johnson

All rights reserved.

ISBN:1979012296
ISBN-13:978-1979012294

DEDICATION

This book is dedicated to all Childhood Cancer Parents.

CONTENTS

	Introduction	i
1	The Concern	Pg. 1
2	The Diagnosis	Pg. 8
3	The News	Pg. 15
4	The Results	Pg. 22
5	The First Chemo	Pg. 26
6	Aunt Gina	Pg. 32
7	The Eviction Notice	Pg. 36
8	Dinosaur Roar	Pg. 43
9	Faith, Prayer, Worship	Pg. 52

INTRODUCTION

On April 3, 2017, our family joined the club that no one wants to be in – the childhood cancer club. We were told that our 19-month-old son David was diagnosed with childhood cancer. I was just a passenger, along for the ride, but I was profoundly affected by the illness that my son had encountered.

I was utterly terrified and shell-shocked at the diagnosis. This book was created to help shed light on the subject of pediatric cancer. Cancer for anyone is never a fair fight. There is a lack of funding for pediatric cancer research. This book will have some happy and sad moments.

I invite you to accompany me as I share the fears, joys, struggles, and triumphs encountered on the ride of a lifetime. Hopefully, this will encourage you to help bring about awareness to Childhood Cancer.

1 THE CONCERN

Hyperemesis gravidarum. That was the diagnosis. My sentence: Five months of bed rest that were a far cry from restful. I was pregnant with my fourth child, a little boy who would have to conquer this horrible rare condition with me. I lost 15 pounds in my first trimester. The vomiting was severe, intense and incessant. But still, the little boy fought on. I was treated constantly for dehydration. The only thing I could stomach was crackers and dry noodles, amid sips of ginger ale. But still, the little boy fought on. I was prescribed several medications, which kept me sedated most of the day. My birth canal was blocked. But through it all, the little boy fought on.

My husband named him David after King David. You see, in the Bible, it was David, a shepherd, who defeated the giant Goliath. He was anointed by God. Our David was facing his own Goliath. He was *our* blessing from God. Following an emergency Caesarean section,

King David emerged – Aug. 10, 2015 – victorious from battle. King David we called him, and the name would stick. As our family celebrated his arrival, we had no idea that another battle would be brewing on the horizon.

****

"You take your children to the doctor for everything," many of my family members would always say. And they were right. If one of my children coughed or sneezed excessively, off we'd go. The trips were so frequent that my family started kidding me about them. Maybe my paranoia was a product of the six years I spent working in a pediatrics office. For it was there that I saw so many illnesses. And I simply didn't want to be caught off guard.

In March 2017, David – my year-old – was running a high fever, and he wasn't getting any better. But kids will be kids, I thought. He was hot to the touch, yet that didn't hinder his playfulness. David had run a high fever a month earlier. At that time, I took him to the nearest children's hospital urgent care center. He was diagnosed with an ear infection, prescribed antibiotics, and sent home. Instead of making my usual dash to the doctor, I held off.

Later that evening, after giving David a bath, I noticed a swelling in his lower abdomen, sort of resembling a football. I called his pediatrician, but she assured me that there was nothing to worry about. She noted that he had just had his 18-month checkup and received a clean bill of health. Still, I had a bad feeling.

Over the next few weeks, David had a growth spurt, but the bulge didn't disappear. "There's something wrong," I told my husband, Rodney. "Don't you think his stomach looks a little big?"

"Stop saying things about it," he said, almost implying that I might be jinxing David. "You're overreacting."

On April Fool's Day, which landed on a Saturday, one of my friends was getting married. I baked a wedding cake for her. David was feverish and irritable at the time. I called his pediatrician, and she recommended I give him Tylenol. I complied, and David's condition improved throughout the day.

The following night, though, the fever returned. I contacted the pediatrician again. She told me to monitor David and bring him to the office on Monday. David's temperature was 104.

The next morning at David's 9 a.m. appointment, the pediatrician looked at his chart. He had not eaten, hadn't drank anything and seemed exhausted. Grasping for answers, the pediatrician said she was unsure what to do. David had yet another ear infection. He had been prescribed three medications, each progressively stronger to combat his symptoms. She said that David might have a urinary tract infection, and that I should take him to the nearest hospital for further testing. I wasn't comfortable with the diagnosis, so I took David to The Children's Hospital of The King's Daughters (CHKD) around noon.

CHKD's emergency room married crisis with a bit of chaos. There were three people in the waiting area. Half of the room was blocked off and under construction. Nonetheless, we were able to be seen at 11 a.m. An emergency room nurse in the check-in area took David's temperature. It was still high. I told her about the recurring ear infections and about the bulge in his belly.

We were then escorted to Triage Room 7, where we were attended to by another nurse. I was asked if I wanted to put David on a stretcher, but he clung tightly to my side, silently insisting that there was where he wanted to be. We proceeded down a hallway lined with painted fish and glossy floors. I insisted they run every test they could to find out what was wrong.

The emergency room physician ordered an X-ray of David's abdomen. We were chaperoned to an area where the procedure was done. The room was dark and the machine was imposing, practically foreboding.

David was strapped into the huge machine. While lying on his back, his arms were restrained above his head to ensure an accurate picture of his abdomen. After the X-rays, we returned to the triage room to await the results. Minutes seemed like an eternity.

After the radiologist noted something on David's left kidney, the emergency room physician wanted a closer look. Meanwhile, my heart raced and concern flooded my face. I thought about my husband. I didn't want to alarm him until we had answers – answers to my questions and to those he might have.

The physician ordered an ultrasound. Within the first 30 minutes of the procedure the technician called another technician into the room. An hour passed, and my anxiety was getting the better of me. I began to ask questions. The technician said she needed to consult with the physician first. There would be more waiting.

I carried David back down the hall to Triage Room 7. It felt like the longest walk ever. I didn't know what to think. I didn't know what to feel. My heart was beating out of my chest. Once we reached the room, I sat there, with David on my lap, Googling for medical diagnoses.

After about a half hour, the door opened. The physician and two residents entered. They asked me to contact my husband and ask him to come to the hospital. They wanted to discuss some things with both of us concerning David. I called Rodney, but didn't get an answer. So I texted him to call me as soon as he could.

Still anxious and scared, I asked to doctor to tell me her prognosis and that I would fill my husband in when he got to the hospital. "I can handle it," I told her. But I would be wrong.

The doctor asked me to sit down. With a look of concern, she uttered four words I'll never forget. "Your son has cancer," she said, sending my world on the verge of spinning out of control.

"What?!?" I rhetorically replied, holding David tightly.

With that I collapsed into tears. I screamed as the doctor futilely attempted to console me. I needed my husband more than anything at that moment. I needed to be able to bury my face in his chest while he held me tight, kissed me on my forehead and told me that everything would be all right. I felt helpless.

Trying to compose myself, I turned my attention to David. "It's OK," I told him, knowing all the while that such was not the case. But that was all I had. He had been diagnosed with a deadly disease, and I was powerless in protecting him from it. My mind was filled with denial. "David was too perfect to have anything wrong with him," I thought.

It took a few minutes for me to gather myself. The physician said there was a large tumor on David's left kidney. It could be one of two cancers: Wilms Tumor or Neuroblastoma. She ordered a CAT scan to get more detailed pictures of the growth.

David was placed on a padded table. He was strapped down again – this time from his chest to his feet. He screamed and yelled for me to pick him up. But I had to let the machine run its course.

Some five hours after arriving at the hospital, David was admitted, and I would stay the night with him. I had prayed for a different result: a checkup, a prescription, a return trip home. But reality erased those options. So many thoughts crossed my mind.

Exhausted emotionally, I still had work to do. It was time to tell Rodney his son wouldn't be coming home that night. It was time to tell him the terrible news. But it wouldn't be easy.

I called him about 5 p.m. and he answered. "What is wrong with my son?" he asked. I pleaded with him to leave work and come to the hospital, but he became increasingly concerned, agitated, and insistent.

"Christina, is my son dying?" he asked. "Tell me my son is not dying."

I broke down. "David has cancer," I relented.

"No," he yelled. "What's really going on?"

2 THE DIAGNOSIS

With my husband still reeling from the somber news, I needed to reach out to other members of the family. My sister, who lived close by, would be first.

"David has cancer," I told her over the phone.

She reacted with disbelief.

"No! What do mean? What do mean? What do you mean he has cancer?" she stammered.

I told her that I didn't have many details yet and that I needed to cut the call short because my phone was dying. I said that we were at The Children's Hospital of the King's Daughters in Norfolk, Va., and that I would get back to her later.

Next, I called my mom. She didn't pick up, so I left her a message letting her know that David was in the hospital and that he would not be coming home for a while. I told her too that my phone was dying and where we were.

I sat in Triage Room 7 sobbing, alone except for

my son who I held tightly in my arms. Compounding my isolation, I also was losing my connection to the outside world through a cell phone that was at less than 15 percent. I looked down at David. Again, I whispered to him that everything would be all right, knowing full well that such was not necessarily the case.

David was only 19 months old. So young, so sweet, so innocent. My son had cancer. My mind began to race, thinking dark thoughts about all the things I might not be able to do with him in his lifetime. At the same time I tried to convince myself that this wasn't happening. It all seemed so surreal. If only I could awake from this nightmare and the sharp pain it inflicted. If only this was not my new reality. My whole world was turned upside down.

After picking up Christiana, our 8-year-old, from school, Rodney raced home and gathered our other two children – Aaliyah, 14, and Blair, 15 – and took them to my grandmother's house. There they would be cared for by my grandmother and Aunt Gina, who lived with her, while Rodney and I sorted things out.

My mom arrived at the hospital that evening around 6:30. She lightly knocked on the door before entering the room. She told me that she had received my message and came straight to the hospital to see what was going on.

She stood there just inside the room with her purse draped over her shoulder and her arms crossed. She bore an expression I hadn't seen before. It was concern mixed with sorrow and confusion. She stared at David in silence. After about 30 minutes filled with awkwardness, she told me to keep her posted and let her know if I needed anything. And then she left.

Around 7 p.m., Rodney arrived, still in his work clothes, and with my phone charger. He, David and I were taken to the eighth floor of the hospital – the hematology and oncology unit. The emergency room physician told us an oncologist was on the way. Our destination: Room 805. The room had a huge barred crib, the sight of which made me realize that this was really happening, and that we wouldn't be sleeping in our own beds that night.

As we waited for the oncologist, I found myself on my phone flipping through old pictures that we had taken. I looked to see if there was something that I might have missed – other symptoms besides the abnormal look of David's tummy. I began to realize that our son's cancer journey had begun, and that soon we would be meeting a team of professionals who would help us care for him.

The oncologist that we saw that night said three things that I will never forget.

"There is nothing that you have done wrong," she said. "There is nothing you could have done; you did not cause this. You did the right thing."

She showed us images of the tumor on the CT scan. She said that it was fairly large and looked as if it stretched from one side of his stomach to the other. She suggested that we get some rest because the next few days were going to be very busy. Several tests would need to be done, she said, and a biopsy of the tumor would need to be performed as soon as possible to figure out what course of action to take. From the looks of the CT scan, she said, she was almost positive it was Neuroblastoma, a childhood cancer found in the small glands on top of the kidneys that can develop in the belly, chest, neck, pelvis and bones. The oncologist assured us that we were in good hands and we would get answers. She informed us that we would be inpatient for the next couple of weeks.

That night of April 3, I feared sleep. I was afraid that if I fell asleep the following morning David would be gone. So I laid next to him and whispered a prayer while he slept. I also found myself researching online the two possible diagnoses that had been given to us, in hopes of finding a silver lining, or at least more information on the cancer.

Every three minutes a child is diagnosed with cancer, I found. I could still hear the words from earlier that day: "Your son has cancer." They were words that shift your world. Words that stick with you forever. Words that made one of my longest nights longer. I wanted so much for David to have surgery to remove the tumor immediately. Unfortunately, that was not possible. The specialists needed more information before they could proceed. We had to wait for the next day to get answers.

I replaced sleep that night with meditation, and pleading to God. I prayed and prayed. A Bible scripture that my grandmother instilled in me as a child came to mind: – Proverbs 3:5-6:

> "Trust in the Lord with all your heart; and lean not to your own understanding, In all your ways acknowledge him, and he shall direct your paths."

I had to look at things through spiritual prism, I told myself. Our world has just changed and there was nothing we could do but put our faith in God's promises. We know that God never changes and he is the same forever more. My husband and I would have to find strength from places that we had never tapped. We would have to allow our flesh to grieve and our spirits to rely on God to take us through this journey.

At long last, the morning came. We got to meet the team of specialists who would be taking care of David and searching for answers. The oncologist on call sat down with us and went over the plan for the next few days. First, doctors would have to get as much information about the tumor as possible.

David's red blood count has dropped below the

normal range, so the oncologist decided that a blood transfusion was needed to prepare him for the next day's surgery. Doing so would make it safer to perform the necessary diagnostic test and procedures that would be needed in the next few days to help develop a concrete treatment plan.

As time arrived for David's surgery, I began wrestling with an important question: When is it OK for you to hand your child over to complete strangers? David would have to go under general anesthesia for the first time. Rodney and I walked him down to the operating room swaddled in one of his favorite blankets. He was given medication to help relax him so it would be an easy transition for him when we surrendered him to the medical team. We would be forced to trust them with the life of our child – one of our most prized possessions.

I watched them carry David down the hall to the operating room. I didn't like that they had to drug him. I stood in the hall with my husband for a few minutes and then we walked to the surgery waiting room. We were given a number that corresponded to David's progress on a screen in the waiting room. I watch patiently for his number to show up and for the board to say "In the operating room." I stared at the board for at least an hour. I felt like crying. I wanted David to be back in my arms. I had to trust that God would protect him during the surgery. I had to trust that with my whole heart. Jesus said: "Cast out all of your cares and I will give you peace." (1 Peter 5:7)

The first procedure that David underwent was a bone marrow biopsy. This test was done to see if the cancer had spread to his bone marrow. The procedure required two small incisions in the buttocks. David also received a small incision near his left kidney to drain fluid that had backed up. Apparently, the tumor was so big that it was causing his kidney to malfunction.

The operation was over, and I was a nervous wreck. I wasn't sure if I was prepared to see how David looked after the operation. When he came to, he cried for us to be there. While I was able pick him up, I noticed that he was attached to a bag – a nephrostomy – which had become a temporary part of him. The nephrostomy provided the means for his kidney to drain.

Looking at my little boy, it was clear that cancer had truly stolen something from us. For the next few months, our child's life would consist of hospital stays surrounded by doctors and nurses. It was time to accept a new normal. He wouldn't be able to go outside and play like other children.

3 THE NEWS

One night, during the first few days at the hospital, I found myself in the bathroom, crying. I dropped my head between my knees, my heart aching, as I wallowed in helplessness. After a few minutes I was able to pull it together, give myself a pep talk and tell myself that I could work through this.

While I stayed at the hospital, the children had been dropped off at my grandmother's house for spring break. I had took a week off to spend with them, but that was no longer possible. Rodney had to return to work, but constantly called seeking results on the tests. Everyone's schedule had been disrupted and rearranged, and all we could do now was brace for updates that couldn't come soon enough.

Every year, millions of children are diagnosed worldwide with a deadly disease. When a child is diagnosed with cancer, the whole family is affected. Getting news that my child had it was already a hard pill to swallow. But one of the most difficult parts of the process was telling my children, his older siblings, that David had been stricken with this deadly disease.

A few days passed, and I could no longer avoid answering the children's questions about why David was not home and why he had to stay in the hospital. We were faced with tough choices. While we knew it would be important to have the children play a role in helping to take care of David when he did get home, it was paralyzing to think of the fear they would face. We would need to educate them about the facts of his condition, yet encourage them to be brave and engage with him. I struggled with my own bravery, but the time had come to tell them. As parents it's impossible to prepare our children for everything that happens in life. However, we can teach them skills to cope in certain situations.

I called my grandmother's house to let the kids know what was going on with David. I didn't know exactly what to say to them, because we weren't sure what the plan for David was going to be. But they kept asking questions and I just couldn't keep them in the dark any longer. I decided to tell Blair and Aaliyah on speaker phone first. When I told them that their brother had cancer, the phone went silent on the other end. I could sense a range of intense emotions. They seemed afraid and anxious.

"Is he OK mom?" Aaliyah asked. "How long do you have to stay there?"

I explained to them that Rodney and I would be at the hospital working on a plan to get David better so that he would be able to come home. As soon as he was better, I told them, we would bring them to the hospital so that they could spend time with him. They knew how serious David's condition was and became extremely concerned. It wasn't the first time that Blair and Aaliyah have heard the "C" word. A boy at our church had been diagnosed with brain cancer. The kids witnessed the flood of prayers that poured out to him every time he was able to attend the service. Still, his condition worsened. His body began to abnormally swell. And one day, the little boy stopped showing up to church. We knew the Lord had taken him.

It wouldn't be any easier to tell Christiana about her little brother's condition. Christiana was David's "little big sister." The two were inseparable. She watched over him like a hawk. When we went to the store, she would be sure to pick something out for him. When it came to snacks, she would make recommendations for the two of them, and then they would sit on David's Mickey Mouse chair and share. When David wasn't feeling well, she would pick him up and comfort him. She would teach David new things and encourage him to say things, as he learned to talk. They even conspired together. Christiana was fiercely loyal to David, coming to his defense in an instant. She loved picking him up and he would rest his head on her shoulder while she rocked him.

I asked Christiana if she knew what cancer was. I could tell by her response that she did not quite understand the severity of his illness. I felt a bit relieved that she did not know about cancer and how it could affect people. I calmly told her that everything would be OK. As those reassuring words creased my lips, a feeling of guilt consumed me. I felt like I had lied to her because

I really did not believe that David was going to be OK. But I did not want her to be sad. I did not want her to shoulder such emotional and psychological issues at such an early age. Then, Christiana uttered a question that tore into my heart:

"Who am I supposed to play with?" she asked.

She said that she wished that this was all over so that she could play with him at home. I assured her that we would let her visit David as often as possible so they could play together while he recovered.

Knowing that the children might feel anxiety, fear, confusion and anger as they tried to cope with David's illness, I urged them to be open about their feelings. We are all in this together, I told them. And with our help, David is going to get well soon, and we will be able to bring him home. I asked them not to tell anyone until we received more test results and worked out a treatment plan for their brother.

"We must have faith that God will bring him through this," I told them. "This is just a test. All we need is a mustard seed of faith."

Faith. Amid my struggle to come to grips with what might lie ahead for David, it was the one word I needed to clutch tightly. It wouldn't be easy though.

Doubt fueled many of my inner battles and I did my best to conceal it in front of the children. I asked them to have faith, even if it was just a little. I asked them to pray to God daily and ask him to heal their baby brother. "We must stick together to get through this," I said. "David will be healed. He will be able to celebrate his second birthday."

There is an extra layer of grief that comes with those who find themselves grief-stricken. If you find yourself the point person in a tragedy, you are forced to relive it again and again as you spread the news to others. This would be my burden as I contacted other family members. For every phone call I made, I had to prepare for the sorrow that will flood from the other end of the phone. I did not want sympathy or special treatment because my son had cancer. I wanted a cure. The hardest part was telling the world. I had to mentally prepare myself for the responses that I would get. I was already overwhelmed with what was happening.

I chose social media, in particular Facebook, to send my message, but Rodney had apparently beaten me to the punch. A torrent of comments had started rolling in already, with people inquiring more about David's condition and what was happening than just sending well-wishes and support. I was already overwhelmed with what was happening. I kept hoping that someone would say something positive like, "All would be well," but that didn't happen. Instead I would hear things like "What stage is his cancer?" "How much time does he have?" or "Did this have something to do with all the complications you had when you were pregnant with him?"

With David on my lap, I responded to the chaos in a Facebook live post. I kept my message simple and direct.

"Some of you may or may not know that King David is in the hospital. We ask that you please be respectful and not overwhelm us with questions while we are trying to seek answers. Please do not just show up at the hospital without talking to us first. Please allow us time to get back with you. … We ask that you pray for our family as we go through this difficult time. We ask that you do not reach out to our relatives and overwhelm them with questions. This eliminates confusion."

Once the word was out, all roads for my husband and I led back to faith. We had to stay strong for King David. We still believed in miracles. My spiritual life before David's diagnosis was already beginning to grow. I was no longer living one day at a time. I lived one hour at a time. Beyond the sorrow, I rejoiced in the Lord for all he had done for me.

April 6, 2017, after three days in the hospital, David received a day of rest. But it would not be without its challenges. He wasn't allowed to eat or drink anything that night. He cried on and off throughout the night because he was not able to have his sippy cup – his source of control and comfort. His struggle became my struggle.

The following day, David had to undergo yet another procedure – this time to insert a catheter in his chest that would allow for IV fluids, antibiotics and chemotherapy. For a second time, we would surrender our son to his treatment team. It would be just as hard as the first time.

The surgery went well, and Rodney and I were reunited with our son in the recovery room. This had been a long week for us. David had endured a battery of tests. Now it was time to await the results, which might take a few days, we were told. But time is a fickle thing. Sometimes there isn't enough time, but in this case there was more time than I needed. My mind remained unsettled, filled with questions. What kind of cancer was it? Had it spread? What were the results? As these dizzying thoughts clouded my mind, the only logical thing Rodney and I could do was pray – and wait.

4 THE RESULTS

As I stared out the hospital window, with David laying on my lap, I imagined him being outside. He should be out there, running around, enjoying the beautiful weather, I said to myself. But the sobering reality was that we were confined to a concrete building, waiting for his test results to come back.

Out in the hallway, to my surprise, there was a red wagon. I decided to take David for a spin in it. But certain measures needed to be observed before the ride. First, David would have to bring his IV with him. That IV pole would become part of David during his hospital stay. No matter where he went, it would stay tethered to him like a shadow. Worst of all, he would have to wear a mask in order to leave the room. The mere sight of the mask made David scream. He didn't want to put it on. I tried distracting him, telling him what fun he would have in the big red wagon. But the ride would fall short of my promises. It would be a lot of work for little return. We were restricted to going in a small circle. There was no new scenery. There was no freedom. Imagination was limited. Just the white walls and hospital room doors reinforcing our confinement.

As I pulled David along in the red wagon, that omnipresent feeling began to sink in again. This was our new normal. We were sentenced to an antiseptic environment, brightened only by pictures of fish on a clock in the room, accented by glossy floors. The sound of IV pumps became normal. Sleep no longer was a priority. Around-the-clock checks for vital signs became commonplace. Having a seriously ill child can be life-altering. It's not something for which you can prepare.

Red wagon aside, there was another special place on the otherwise character-less floor: The playroom down the hall. The playroom was sanitized from top to bottom, and children would have to sanitize their hands before entering. There, David could meet other children who were also burdened with IV poles.

Nonetheless, David loved the playroom. It was the happiest place in the hospital. Its brightly colored walls with ABC and 123 banners added to the frolicsome atmosphere. There were comfortable couches to sit on. There were video games. There was even a play kitchen, which David favored most. He loved to cook and enjoyed pretending to crack a toy egg to make a cake. There also was a huge rug where we would sit for music time every Thursday.

Adjoining the playroom was an enclosed patio, which on

nice days was an ideal place for David to go. The patio was equipped with a play set with tunnels and slides, David's favorite. He would navigate them as best he could with his IV in tow. The patio was often times restricted because of humid spring days.

Also restricted was the playroom in general, which had set hours. When it was closed, David would throw fits. He would fall on the floor, crying and saying, "I want to go to the playroom." Despite me repeating that the playroom was closed, he would remain inconsolable.

Rodney and I found ourselves inconsolable as well during our wait for answers. Repeatedly, we asked the hospital staff for the test results. The moment the doctor would crack open the door, we would pounce in our quest for news. Our inquiries reached a point that when the doctor would walk in, he would quickly fire off, "We are just checking in; no results yet," to keep us at bay.

After what seemed like an eternity, one of the test results came back. David did not have cancer in his bone marrow, the doctor said. The cancer resided in one local area and hadn't spread. I took a deep breath in relief. But the wait wasn't over. Rodney and I still awaited the results of the biopsy, which would determine the course of treatment.

While we waited, nurses began grooming us on how to care for our son. Once regular exercises would have to be modified. Because of David's nephrostomy bag, he wouldn't be able to take a bath. "How crazy is that?" I thought. "Every kid loves to splash and play in the water."

The following day, a team of doctors entered our room. It was time. The final results were in. My face was drenched in concern, and my palms began to sweat, as I sat next to Rodney. One doctor sat on the edge of the bed with papers in his hands. He started discussing David's condition using medical jargon that I found as confusing as it was elusive. My reaction was the interrupt him.

"Can you just tell me what it is?" I asked impatiently. I had waited long enough.

"It is Neuroblastoma," the doctor replied.

He then gave us the results with the measurements of the tumor. Fortunately, the tumor was only on David's left kidney. My relief was still mixed with anxiety and a dose of fear though. I smiled at Rodney.

"Praise God," he responded. We were now ready to develop a treatment plan for David.

5 THE FIRST CHEMO

When you receive news that your child has cancer, you immediately become an advocate for your child. The battle had begun for Rodney and I, and we had a difficult journey ahead of us. I found myself looking at a handout that one of the nurses gave us right after the diagnosis. It was bright yellow with beautiful colors. At the top of the handout were these dreaded words: "Childhood Cancer Roadmap." There was an extensive checklist, detailing the arduous process toward recovery. We were able to check off the first item: "test and diagnosis."

As David and I stared out the hospital window, I longed for him to be outside running around and enjoying the beautiful weather. It nearly broke my heart that he was trapped in a hospital room that had now become our second home.

Because of the pressure being put on David's kidney by the tumor, he had developed high blood pressure. He was prescribed daily medication to keep his pressure stable. One of the doctors recommended inserting a feeding tube in David in case he rejected taking his medication and stopped eating. While I'm not one usually to question or complain about a doctor's suggestions, the thought of a feeding tube made me uneasy – especially given that David was taking his meds and eating.

When the doctor entered the room with the consent form for the feeding tube, Rodney and I got very upset. We didn't see the need, and refused to sign it, despite the doctor's pleas. The doctor left the room with the form unsigned, but soon after another doctor arrived. He explained to us the benefits of the feeding tube, but his words were falling on deaf ears. A feeding tube was out of the question, we told the doctor. We also cautioned him on sending anyone else to try to convince us to allow the procedure. As far as we were concerned, David hadn't loss any weight and if he did, we would cross that road when we got to it. As a result of our continued objections, the doctors relented and David's treatment continued without the feeding tube.

About a week later, Rodney and I decided to allow visitors to come to the hospital. We would allow immediate family members and our church's pastor. Initial reactions were filled with sorrow, but once we took each visitor aside individually and testified about our optimism and God's healing power, their sadness transformed into happiness. "David is going to be all right; he's in God's hands," we told them. Pastor David from our church dropped in to see David. "This is a test for my wife and I," Rodney told him, smiling confidently. "This will be for God's glory because David is already healed."

The following week, we decided it was a good time to bring the siblings to the hospital to see him. Social workers at the hospital encouraged us to allow the older children to be involved in caring for David. This would allow for a smooth transition once David was discharged, they said. Rodney picked up the children from my grandmother's house and brought them to the hospital. As I watched the door slowly crack open to our hospital room, Blair peered from behind it first. I could tell by the look on his face that he didn't know that to expect. He seemed at once sad, yet concerned. "Look David, your brother Blair is here," I said happily. David sat up. "Hey bear!" he responded. Blair began to smile and relax a little, as the girls walked in slowly behind him. Their faces lit up when they saw that David was active and smiling. David showed them all his toys he had got from the hospital, and also went with them to the playroom. Blair and Aaliyah weren't sure how to hold David because he was attached to the bag, but we showed them how to pick him up and how to hold the bag at the same time. Later, we found a Spiderman backpack that we put his tubing and bag in so David didn't step on it while playing.

When Christiana first saw David, she was afraid. She stared at the bag attached to him for a long time. She asked if it hurt when he got the IV. I told her that her brother was brave and that she should continue to pray for him. They gave each other a hug and David instantly wanted to show her some of the things he did at the hospital. He showed her all the toys that he had gotten. At that moment, it was as if no time had passed between the two. They picked up where they left off.

Chemotherapy. The time had come. A nurse educator sat down with Rodney and I and provided details of what to expect following David's first treatment. Side effects differed from patient to patient we learned. Besides hair loss, one common side effect is mucositis. This causes white sores in your mouth. And there is nausea. We were warned that the treatment could result in vomiting.

David's vitals were taken, several nurses entered the room, and one of them hung a small clear bag on his IV pole that had liquid in it.

"Where is the chemo medication?" I asked.

"It is right here in this clear bag," the nurse replied.

I was expecting chemicals with frightening labels, but it wasn't scary at all. Rodney and I stared at the IV pump as we waited for the nurse to start the infusion. I watched as the first drop dripped slowly from the IV chamber. The nurses stayed in the room for the first few minutes to make sure David didn't have an adverse reaction to the medication.

We waited, staring at David to see what was going to happen next. Would he throw up or experience a high fever? Those were possibilities, we were told. But a few hours later and nothing happened. The first dose of chemo was successfully completed and there was no immediate reaction. However, our optimism was tempered by the expectation of delayed side effects that could surface in the next 10 days when David's blood count would plummet.

While chemotherapy is used to kill cancer cells, science still hasn't figured out a way to make it exclusively kill cancer cells. It kills all cells. One side effect of the treatment is hair loss – not just the hair on your head, but your eyebrows, eye lashes and arm pit hair. All hair. A few days passed after the treatment, and still no fever or hair loss. David's blood count had dropped to zero, so we were put in isolation. David couldn't leave the room. The waiting game returned: This time for his blood counts to rebound so we could go home. The whole ordeal had been more than three weeks old and Rodney and I were running low on energy and running empty on patience. During our wait, we received education on how to care for David at home. We were assigned a social worker from the hospital to assist us with resources for families dealing with cancer.

After four weeks, we were released to go home. Another checkbox on the roadmap was checked off. Rodney went ahead of David and I to make sure the house was extra clean. We didn't want to take any chances of him getting sick. When we got home I felt so at peace. I was finally able to sleep in my own bed.

I bathed David the following day. As I combed his hair, I realized his hair was coming out in the comb. The side effects were finally happening. I called Rodney at work. "He's all right," Rodney said. "Don't panic."

But I wasn't ready to see how David would look without hair. I broke down for the second time, this time with David in my arms. He just patted me on the back, as I held him tightly and told him, "mommy is okay and you are going to be all right."

By the end of the day most of his hair was gone. I decided not to shave the remaining wisps on his head because I was afraid that it might hurt. When his siblings got home from school, David was sleep. I told them that David lost his hair. I told them he would look a little different, but not to panic.

6 AUNT GINA

Two days after David's first treatment, we had an appointment at the oncology clinic for a checkup. When we walked in we met Rob, David's primary nurse. Nurse Rob would be caring for David throughout his treatment. Nurse Rob was a white male in his 30s, about 5'7" with brown hair. He was very tender and compassionate and guided us through our first day at the clinic. He took the time to explain everything and took extra precautions when caring for David. He stayed in the room when the doctors came to visit and always asked if we had any questions. He was very transparent and honest. He told us that there would be a lot of highs and lows. He would advocate for us. If we needed anything, don't hesitate to call, he said. Nurse Rob was like a favorite uncle.
The clinic walls were filled with color, and the floors were painted with sea creatures. As we walked down the long hall to go to the back of the clinic, there was a playroom. The playroom was amazing, and David was eager to go play with the other kids, who like him were stricken with this horrible disease.

During David's second inpatient treatment in May, I received a call from my sister telling me that I needed to come to the hospital immediately. It was Aunt Gina. She was in intensive care and it wasn't known whether or not she would recover. Rodney watched David while I raced frantically across town to meet the rest of the family at the hospital. Reaching speeds of 80 mph, I screamed in my car as I barreled down the highway. "God, what now? Why is this happening?"

I felt like I was at my breaking point. I was enrolled fulltime at school, working, and taking care of David at the same time. And now this. I felt my heart drop again. I knew that God would not put more on me than I could bear, but I was still feeling emotionally overwhelmed. Aunt Gina was always there for the family. She watched over my children and they loved her dearly.

When I arrived at the hospital, the family was gathered in the waiting room. I stopped there. They were consumed in hopelessness and sorrow. I went to Aunt Gina's room. She was hooked up to machines and surrounded by IV poles. She had about six of them. It reminded me a little of David during inpatient treatment, but worse. The sight scared me. Her body was shutting down.

The doctors told us that they are going to try to do surgery to see if they would be able to save her. This occurred the week of my graduation from college. Aunt Gina had watched my children for several years while I attended night classes toward my degree. I couldn't imagine her being absent from my commencement. She needed to be there. But there she was, sedated with tubes everywhere, more tubes than I had ever seen. I leaned over and whispered in her ear that everything would be all right and that she was going to fight this. Deep down inside, though, I knew that the end might be near for her.

When I got home, I told the kids that Aunt Gina was sick, but I could not muster up the strength to tell them how sick she was. I decided to wait until after the surgery before I gave them more information.

Graduation day came, but it arrived with a dose of gloom. I should have been excited, but I wasn't. Most of the family members who were going to attend my graduation were at the hospital with Aunt Gina, who was supposed to be there as well. Inside, I was angry. Before the commencement ceremony I found myself sitting on the bathroom floor crying out to God, looking for guidance, strength and help. I finally got up and wiped my tears. God had bigger plans for me, I told myself. I needed to go through with this and keep it together.

David was just discharged from his second round of chemotherapy the day before my graduation. He would stay home with Rodney. My mom drove the other children to the ceremony, while I arrived ahead of time. Today I would put on my best smile, but it wouldn't be easy. My husband, my baby boy and my Aunt Gina would be absent. Aunt Gina, who believed in me. Aunt Gina, who pushed me. I said a prayer as I walked across the stage. I did it! I graduated. The past six weeks of school were the most difficult, but I made it through with God's help. After graduation, I got another troubling call from the hospital. Aunt Gina wasn't going to make it. My hand was forced. I had to tell the kids the truth. I told them that she was not doing well and that we needed to go to the hospital. I asked if they wanted to go and they said they did.

When we arrived at the hospital, I was still dressed in my cap and gown. I walked Aaliyah and my niece Naomi back to see Aunt Gina. As soon as we entered the room, Naomi and Aaliyah collapsed on the floor. I held them and told them that things would be OK. But things were not OK. Aunt Gina was dying. Aaliyah told her how much she loved her before we left the room. Her words weighed on my heart. While I was crossing the stage, Aunt Gina had been fighting for her life. She lost that fight later that night. It was May 13, 2017, a bittersweet day I'll never forget.

7 THE EVICTION NOTICE

David successfully completed two rounds of chemotherapy with minimal side effects. During his treatments, he would roam the hospital halls, becoming very comfortable with the nurses. At night, nurses would look forward to seeing David because he would come out his room from time to time into the nurses' pod and dance for them.

Round three of chemotherapy would prove much more difficult than the first two treatments. Rodney and I were told to expect David to be sick to his stomach. Within the first 15 minutes of the treatment, David began vomiting. I began to worry. The hospital staff kept us calm by checking on us frequently. They had medications on standby and were very supportive. I felt like this would be David's biggest hurdle. He was confined to a hospital bed. There would be no dancing, no playing. Just cuddles from Rodney and I.

The next two rounds were a breeze. David was doing amazing. It was July and time for surgeons to safely remove as much of the tumor as they could. David's birthday was the following month so we decided to do his 2-year-old photos early as well as his birthday party. The theme was Disney and the atmosphere was festive. Family members and church members packed my mother's yard. We invited Mickey Mouse as well as a DJ to help celebrate. David and his siblings danced the day away. It was as if things had returned to normal.

Two days later, the sobering reality returned. It was time for us to head to the hospital for David's surgery. I was happy at the prospect of removing the tumor, yet nervous about to possibility that something could go wrong. I tossed and turned the night before. I couldn't sleep a wink. Before I knew it, it was 5 a.m. and time to go.

Rodney and I packed the car, grab David's giant Mickey Mouse doll as well as our suitcase, and off we went. Rodney prayed for the hospital staff as well as the others during the drive. "He is healed already, Lord," he prayed. "Allow the surgeons to remove the tumor with no other obstacles. Protect his organs in the process."

As we pulled into the hospital it hit me. Our baby would be going under the knife, having major surgery. He was going to be sedated for a few hours during the procedure and Rodney and I would not be there in the operating room with him. Instead of comforting him, we would face the discomfort of anxiety and fear as we awaited the outcome. The whole scenario sent a chill through me.

While waiting for the nurses to take him to the operating room, David fell asleep in my arms. I felt a bit of relief that he was sleeping, hopeful that it would make the transition easier when we had to hand him off to the hospital staff. During our wait Pastor David came by to pray for David.

On pins and needles, we prepared to give David to the medical staff. As we approached them, I observed them checking to make sure they appeared to be well rested and focused. I wanted to make sure that he was in good hands. To my surprise, David did not throw a fit during the exchange. I figured he was still exhausted from all the excitement of the birthday party.

Pastor David sat with us in the surgery waiting room, in hopes of bringing peace and comfort to Rodney and I. His presence kept our minds off what was going on. Then, about 30 minutes later, the waiting room phone rang.

"Will the parents of David come to the front; I have an update for you," the receptionist said.

She handed the phone to me and the nurse on the other end said that everything was going well and David was doing great. We will update you in the next hour, she said.

I shared the news with my husband and Pastor David. Then I returned to my newly adopted pastime: watching the clock. My attempts to will those hands of time to move faster were futile. Whenever the phone would ring, my heart would jump. Finally, the call came in.

The nurse said that they were done with surgery and David was on his way to the recovery room. The surgeon would be out in a few minutes to talk with us, she said.

Shortly thereafter, David's surgeon walked into the waiting room. Everything looks good, he said. He said he removed a lot of the tumor, but part of it could not be safely extracted. While we had been told initially that David might lose part or all of his kidney, the doctor said that his kidney was left undisturbed. He also told us that they had to insert a tube through David's nose cavity to help drain fluid and that David would not be able to eat for few days while his stomach settled from the surgery.

Pastor David departed, and Rodney and I headed to see David in the recovery room. Seeing David with a nose tube made me a bit uneasy. When I saw David, I cried inside. I rubbed his head and told him that everything would be OK.

The nurses showed me his scar. David was cut across his stomach, from one side to the other. The scar reminded me of the one that remained from the emergency C-section I underwent as the doctor worked to save David during childbirth. I asked permission to hold him and did so ever so delicately for fear of hurting him. Rodney, bearing a look of concern, seemed a bit nervous when I passed David to him. He asked the nurse how long David would have to have the tube in his nose. The nurse replied that it would be for a couple days.

Regardless, David was determined to do something about the tube. He started tugging at it, but it was taped down pretty well, so he initially was unable to dislodge it. Rodney and I warned the nurse that David wouldn't give up that easy.

We stayed in the recovery room for about an hour before being transferred to the intensive care unit (ICU), where David could be monitored closely. The room was smaller and it had a clear large door. It felt as if we were in a cage being observed. When we reached the ICU, David was asleep. A nurse placed him in a barred crib. David was receiving morphine through a pump to help control any pain he might have.

We stood close by and watched him as he slept. It wouldn't be long before we both plopped down and drifted off to sleep as well. When we awoke, David had pulled the tube out of his nose. The nurses insisted that it needed to go back in. A nurse came in and stuck the tube back in his nose, with David fighting all the way. I was livid. I thought perhaps they should have numbed the area before re-inserting the tube. I grabbed David and held him tight, comforting him until he dozed off.

Meanwhile, Rodney left the ICU for a moment to gather himself. The ICU was a bit much for him. There were sick children everywhere. Monitors beeped incessantly. We were not allowed to close the door or cut the lights on. It was unnerving to say the least.

I was able to put David back in the crib while I attempted to get some sleep. I was awakened suddenly by David, who had pulled the tube out of his noise again and this time he was trying to get out of the crib. I called the nurse and told her that we were not going to let them re-insert the tube. I advised her to document it if she wanted.

"No, we are not doing that," I said. "If he needs it, then you're going to have to put him to sleep to do it, but not while he is awake."

In no time at all, David was ready to dance again. "Mommy, I want to go to the playroom," he said.

"David, you just had major surgery," I replied. "Let's just relax, OK?"

That wasn't the answer David was looking for, so a battle of wills ensued. Rodney and I spent the night trying to keep him distracted, because he wanted to get down and walk. David, ever resilient, didn't appear to be experiencing any soreness or pain.

"Nothing can stop King David," Rodney said. "He's ready to go home."

8 DINOSAUR ROAR

The following morning we were transferred to Room 8B. Initially, we were supposed to spend a few days in the intensive care unit, but because of David's speedy recovery we were transferred to a regular room. As we headed to the room, David's favorite place in the hospital caught his eye.

"I want to go to the playroom," he said. "It's open."

Given all that David had been through, it seemed like a good idea, so we let him get out of the bed and walk. Almost instantly, he started dancing. When the surgeon dropped by to visit David, he was mystified. He didn't hesitate to express his disbelief.

"Wow! He's already up and moving?" he said. "Didn't we just do surgery on this kid?"

Resolutely, Rodney replied that not even surgery could put King David down. I was about to find out just how correct he was.

I spent the next few days chasing after David as he played. His energy seemed endless. He could not keep still. After four days in Room 8B, we were allowed to go home – temporarily. After a few weeks of recovery, David would have to return for two rounds of high-dose chemotherapy. Then, he would have to undergo a stem cell transplant using cells harvested from him at the beginning of his treatment.

***

It was Aug. 31, 2017. We had done a ton of packing. It was necessary. We had to be prepared to spend as many as 30 days in the hospital. And it wouldn't be easy for any of us.

High-dose chemotherapy has its own set of protocol and intangibles. I carefully read each form I was given that listed potential side effects. David was put in an isolated room to ensure close monitoring while his medication was administered. He also was hooked up to a blood oxygen monitor, which required him to be tethered to several wires that would restrict his movement.

Some of the reactions we had to watch for were pretty scary. We were told one medication could possibly cause David's skin to burn and peel. We were instructed to bathe him with only water four times a day. We had to be careful when picking him up not to get the medication on us, because it could burn our skin as well. David insisted on being cuddled after the treatment. So I took the risk to comfort him.

A day after David's treatment, he was prepped for his first stem cell transplant. I battled emotions about the procedure. The word transplant was as frightening as some of the possible chemo side effects. After the high dose of chemo, David's white blood cell count had dropped, which meant three things. First, David's immune system was severely compromised. Second, he would have to be kept in isolation. And third, anyone visiting him would be required to carefully wash their hands and wear a yellow suit and mask to prevent transferring harmful germs to him.

The transplant actually wasn't as bad as I thought. A bag on his IV pole contained his stem cells in it. With a nervous stare, Rodney and I watched as the first drop dripped into the IV chamber to be injected in David. We continued our stare, waiting for a reaction from David. Nothing. The room began to smell like creamed corn. I believed the bag was where the odor emanated. The transplant, which proved successful, lasted for about 30 minutes.

I remained at the hospital for another week as we waited for David's blood count to rebound. David was confined to the room, so I downloaded some fun apps on his tablet that he had grown to love. On Sept. 19, we were finally discharged. As we headed down the hallway en route to freedom, we were showered with confetti in celebration of David completing his treatment.

David's final chemotherapy treatment started exactly a month later. King David had weathered the storm of treatments and this was to be his final one. As he received his first medication, there was no reaction – all was well. However, the next infusion caused his right eye and lips to start swelling. The chemo had to be halted, and David was given some Benadryl and held under observation for a few hours.

When his eye and lips began to return to normal, David was given a long-acting steroid to prevent any flare-up. The doctor discontinued the treatment and sent us home for a week, promising to discuss further treatment. When we returned, David was given the first medication he received in the previous treatment. As with the first time, there was no side effect.

The day we had long awaited had finally come. We celebrated as David headed home after his final chemo treatment. It was a milestone. It was a victory. But it wasn't a cure. The threat of cancer still held our hopes hostage. Radiation was the next step.

In stride, we cherished our three weeks of freedom from the hospital. We took it easy, knowing that more treatment lie ahead.

On Oct. 12, 2017, Rodney and I met with the radiation team to go over the next part of David's treatment. It was decided that David would receive radiation treatments at Norfolk General Hospital because it was the closest location. He would have to be sedated to administer the radiation. It would be important for him to remain still during treatments so that the radiation wouldn't go to any other areas of his body and cause harm to any major organs. The treatment had to be the same day at the same time, which meant that we would be going to the hospital Monday through Friday for treatment.

We got a call from the pre-admissions department letting us know that David's scheduled radiation time would be at 1:00 p.m., which would interfere with his routine. Since he was going to be put to sleep, we had to abide by certain cut-off times for eating and drinking. Rodney and I became extremely concerned. We asked the nurses to talk to the anesthesiologist to see if radiation treatment could be moved up. After numerous of calls and complaints, we were able to move his cut-off time.

As for the radiation treatments, we found out that David would need to have 20 rounds of radiation instead of the 15 we were told initially. We had been hoping that the treatments would be finished by Thanksgiving. But there would be no such chance now. Rodney had to work, so for the first treatment it would just be David and I. I was anxious about being alone in the waiting area. At least when I was with Rodney I could talk to him and keep my mind off things. I feared the potential places my mind would roam – as I sat there alone.

David awoke in a good mood the first day of radiation. His energy was contagious. We are going to have a good day I thought to myself, we arrived at CHKD around 10:30 a.m. to get checked in. We were now ready to go over to Norfolk General, and took a tunnel connecting CHKD to the hospital. David did not want to ride on a stretcher so I carried him. The halls were mustard yellow and gave off a depressing vibe. Norfolk General was an adult hospital so there were no bright fish on the floor, no artwork on the walls, nothing that produced a sense of joy. Just mustard yellow walls. I was happy that we were close to the end of treatment, yet sad that David still had to endure this next phase of treatments. My nerves were on edge, even though I was told what to expect. David had been put to sleep several times before, but it still felt like the first time. I found myself again entrusting my son to a group of strangers.

The medical team escorted us to the room where David would receive his treatment. In the hallway on the wall was a brass bell with a rope attached. Once David finished all of his treatments, he would get to ring the bell. The thought of him doing so warmed my heart.

The medical team at Norfolk General Hospital was ready for us. I sat with David on the stretcher so that the anesthesiologist could give him some medicine to make him relax. They called it "happy juice." The medicine was delivered through David's IV as I held him in my arms. Once he was out, I laid him across an operating table and surrendered him to the medical team. I took one last look at the radiation machine and prayed that there wouldn't be any malfunctions. I was then escorted out the room to the waiting area.

I sat there in silence and waited alone. The next 10 minutes felt like eternity. They rolled a still sleeping David out of the treatment room on a stretcher to be reunited with me. The nurses said he did great. Because David was under anesthesia, he had a monitor attached to his bed. We were shuttled back to CHKD, where he would recover.

As we walked down the halls of CHKD, some of the hospital workers cleared the way for us as we drew near. Looks of concern flooded their faces as we passed. We arrived to the recovery area and I was allowed to be by David's side the whole time. With a loud roar, David awoke. The commotion made all the nurses laugh. David tried to sit up but was still a bit woozy from the anesthesia. He asked for a red popsicle while he emerged from the medically induced fog. The roar and popsicle became a routine for the remaining 19 treatments. On Fridays, we would play the "Ice Cream and Cake" song, and all the nurses would gather and dance with David. He was the sunshine on a cloudy day for those around him. His energy was infectious.

David successfully completed all 20 rounds of radiation. The nurses said that they were going to miss his dinosaur roar and things wouldn't be the same without him. They said they would carry on the Friday tradition of the "Ice Cream and Cake" song.

A week after David's radiation treatments, Rodney and I noticed during bath time that he had a long black burn on his spine. The side effects from the radiation treatment were finally showing up. I called the nurse to inform them the day before David's clinic appointment. She confirmed that it was one of the side effects and it eventually would disappear.

Next up for David was immunotherapy treatment. It would consist of five cycles of therapy. This meant that we had to stay at the hospital for four days for each treatment. The first treatment would be in the intensive care unit. Some of the side effects included low blood pressure, fluid retention, and high fevers. The ICU was my least favorite place.

The first round went well. David ran a high fever, but he responded to the treatment well. We got three weeks off before returning to the hospital. This time he received the treatment in room 8B.

For the second cycle, he was given a different medication. The first and second days went well, but on the third day, David started screaming when he went to the bathroom. His groin area had swollen. It looked like he had blood in his diaper. Every time he would urinate, he would scream and yell. I immediately called the nurse. The doctors were called and they ran tests, but nothing came back. David continued to cry as his groin continued to swell. None of the treatments were working. I frantically requested other specialists to examine David. After a day of complaining, a urologist came to see David. He was given a topical medication that produced positive results. David was feeling better. We later found out that David had been suffering from a urine imbalance that was causing extra fluid to build up in his groin area. Because of his condition, we were forced to spend an extra day at the hospital for monitoring.

The third round was also in 8B. It went as smoothly as the first round. The fourth round was a bumpy ride though. It took place in the ICU as an extra precaution. When the treatment began, David's blood pressure started to rise. The treatment was halted for a several minutes. When it resumed, his blood pressure spiked again. This time it was dangerously high. Rodney and I insisted that the treatment be stopped. The doctors tried to convince us to continue but we declined. The following day we were discharged from the hospital.

9 FAITH, PRAYER, WORSHIP

April 21, 2018, was a big day for David. The Roc Solid Foundation was building a playset for him in our backyard. The Chesapeake-based foundation, whose mission is to "build hope for families facing pediatric cancer," prepares "ready bags," which contain provisions needed during unexpected hospital stays. At the time of David's diagnosis, we received a ready bag. The foundation also builds playsets for children age 1-8 and completes top-to-bottom room makeovers for children ages 8-18. Today the foundation would not only treat us to breakfast and a short getaway, but it would construct the playset at our home in our absence.

The foundation's limousine pulled up to our house at about 8:30 that morning. As David, Rodney, and I – along with the immediate family, my mom, and my son's girlfriend -- walked out of the front door, volunteers from the foundation lined up to greet David and usher us to the limousine. The sheer size of the car intimidated David, who clung to Rodney as we approached it. Once inside, David was somewhat relieved. Outside, the volunteers cheered us as we departed. The interior of the limo was colorful and glittery. David speechlessly inspected the unfamiliar surroundings. "It's like a train," we told him.

Our first destination was a Cracker Barrel in Chesapeake. It was as if we were celebrities. Patrons in front of the restaurant gawked in wonderment of who would exit the limo. Once inside, David requested pancakes and bacon. After Cracker Barrel, we had a choice of taking David wherever he wanted. King David chose Chuck E. Cheeses.

At about noon, we headed for home. As we pulled in front of our house, the foundation volunteers as well as some of our family members had gathered to greet David. A television news crew was also on hand, gathering every moment – from us stepping out of the limo to our journey to the backyard. Again, David held Rodney tight, uncertain of what was going to happen next. When we finally reached the end of the sidewalk and opened the gate, family members had gathered around the new playset, smiles adorning their faces. The expression on David's face was priceless. His eyes widened with a mixture of "Wow" with "Why?" It took him a minute to take it all in. While David soaked in the scene, big sister Christiana decided to give the playset a test drive. David followed.

We held a small ceremony for David, thanking everyone for making the moment so special. Rodney and I cried tears of joy as we told the volunteers how thankful we were to have a great day out with no stress and worry, and how the moment reminded us of how our lives were before David's diagnosis.

Our little boy had a brand new playset. He now was able to play outside in the safe confines of home.

Our busy morning turned into a busy day. Rodney and I did three interviews that day – two with local TV news channels and one with the local newspaper. The bustle and excitement of the day left us exhausted.

Once everyone was off to bed, we gave David his nightly medications and he, Rodney and I sprawled out on the bed. As we relaxed, David began complaining that his eye itched. At first, Rodney said David must have something in his eye. I suspected that it was a reaction to his medicine.

A few minutes later David's eyes started swelling. Rodney tried washing his face, but the swelling persisted. Then his lips started to swell. "It's got to be an allergic reaction," I yelled, quickly shifting to panic mode. I dashed downstairs and grabbed the Benadryl out of David's diaper bag. In the seconds it took me to return, David's tongue had begun swelling as well. He started screaming and rocking uncontrollably. He grabbed his chest.

Rodney and I stood there frozen momentarily.

Then I belted out, "CALL 911, NOW!"

While Rodney tried to calm David down, I gave him the Benadryl and grabbed the phone from Rodney. It seemed like the phone rang forever before the operator picked up. The operator answered the phone.

"What's your emergency?" she asked.

"My 2-year-old son, who is a cancer patient, is having an allergic reaction," I said. I explained to the operator David's symptoms, and she asked me to hold on the line until she could contact a paramedic. As I waited, seconds seemed like minutes.

I looked over at Rodney and grabbed David. Rodney was in shock. I asked him to grab some items for David, anticipating that we would be rushed to the hospital. When the ambulance arrived about 15-20 minutes later, Rodney was still in shock – he was frozen, just standing there.

This was David's first ride in an ambulance, and I was hoping for a short, speedy trip. I helped attached his car seat to an awaiting stretcher as my patience dwindled. I chose to ride with David to the hospital. I instructed Rodney – who was still paralyzed standing outside the ambulance – to grab some things and meet us there. When we arrived at the hospital, it was confirmed that David had had an allergic reaction. We were released two hours later and got home about 4 a.m. In an effort to avoid another allergic reaction episode, we gave David Benadryl with his medications.

Fortunately, David's fifth and final cycle of immunotherapy went as smooth as his first and third treatments. Rodney and I breathed a sigh of relief. King David and battled adversity and triumphed, we believed. We were proud of him and we counted our blessings.

I believe the best part of a church service is testimony time. That's when you get to hear all the good news. God has blessed or healed someone. Psalms 66:16 says, "Come and hear, all ye that fear God, and I will declare what he hath done for my soul." During David's treatments, weekly church testimonies gave me an opportunity to share what God was doing in our lives. It also gave our family an opportunity to provide hope to others. While David wasn't able tell others what he had been through, I bore witness to God's power in our son's life.

Before David's journey, I never thought I would have been able to handle it mentally. However, God says that he would not put anything on us that we cannot bear. He prepares us in advance for the storms we may face. He equips us with the tools ahead of time that may be necessary for our battle. It is up to us on whether we use them or not. Among the greatest tools are Faith, Prayer, and Worship.

Why did God choose me? I have no answer. Why wouldn't he choose me?

One valuable thing that I gained during this journey was support from strangers who became our closest friends. I have met some amazing parents who are also on a journey similar to ours.

You never know how God will use you. We had the honor sharing our story on the radio. Keeping busy seemed to help me cope during this journey. It was hard to concentrate on just one thing at the time. I faced a real tough reality: Outside of prayer, there was nothing I could do to change David's diagnosis. I often stopped and took deep breaths and held self-pep talks just to get through the day.

I learned that blood does not make a person family, and that sometimes the people you think won't be there for you, are there for you. And those people are real family. I learned to live in the moment, while being prepared for an unexpected future. Things can change, I learned – and do so rapidly.

It hard for me to wrap my brain around how far we have come and how our family has changed through this journey. We no longer take life for granted. The little things count. The reality is, this could happen to any child. Cancer doesn't discriminate.

In a way, King David has slayed his giant. Through it all, he danced and played. He never stop fighting and we never stopped praying and speaking positively about his life. Although David's journey is not over, he has endured all the pain and suffering with the help of God. This battle was beyond our control and we had to allow God to see us through it. We survived it, and it has strengthened us. And we are still fighting for King

David!

www.ingramcontent.com/pod-product-compliance
Lightning Source LLC
Chambersburg PA
CBHW050017230526
45470CB00003B/1010